Spiritual Warrior
One Man's Cancer Journal

*Only as a (spiritual) warrior can one withstand the path
of knowledge. A warrior cannot complain or regret
anything. His life is an endless challenge and challenges
cannot possibly be good or bad. Challenges are simply
challenges. The basic difference between an ordinary
man and a warrior is that a warrior takes everything as
a challenge, while an ordinary man takes everything as a
blessing or a curse.*

- from the teachings of Don Juan
by Carlos Castaneda

by Dan Blasutti

Foreword and Introduction by Judy Blasutti
Afterword by Pat Carty

Spiritual Warrior
One Man's Cancer Journal

Publication made possible by
Manulife Financial, Waterloo, Ontario

ISBN 0-9681262-0-0

First Canadian Edition
Printed in Canada by Twin City Dwyer Printing Co. Ltd.
Published by The Luce Press, Kitchener, Ontario

The publisher and HopeSpring Cancer Support Centre gratefully acknowledge
the support of Manulife Financial.

Front Cover Photograph by John McEachen
Inside sketches and sculptures by Dan Blasutti
Sketches enhanced by Laura Tindall

Dedicated to all whose path leads to HopeSpring Cancer Support Centre

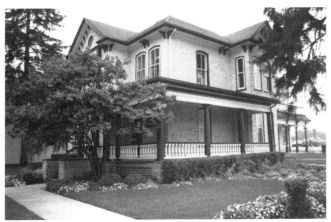

HopeSpring Cancer Support Centre opened in the fall of
1995 at 167 King Street South, Waterloo, Ontario.

HopeSpring Cancer Support Centre was founded to meet the
emotional and spiritual needs of cancer patients and those
who support them. Having cancer himself, Dan Blasutti
recognized the great need for this type of support in his
community and was a member of the HopeSpring
Board of Directors when he died.

CONTENTS

ACKNOWLEDGEMENTS

Thanks to special friends and family who have been on the journey with us. Throughout Dan's illness we were blessed with the love and support of so many.

Thanks to Dan's colleagues and friends at Manulife Financial; big company, big heart.

Thanks to the team who worked with me to publish this book. I wish to thank especially Pat Carty and Betty Recchia from HopeSpring; Brian VanNorman, teacher and writer; John Varden, freelance editor; Phillip Bast, entertainment editor for The Kitchener-Waterloo Record; Irene Gesza, publisher of WholeLife Magazine; and Brad Blain, Director of the Kitchener-Waterloo Art Gallery. From Manulife Financial, special thanks to John Salmond, Shelley Livock, Angela Weller and Tony Niederer.

FOREWORD

There is a crack in everything.
That's how the light gets in.[1]
-Leonard Cohen -

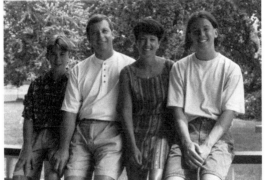

Michael, Dan, Judy, Dennis

Photo: Mark Shea

My husband Dan Blasutti died on Thursday, October 5, 1995 of cancer. He was 41 years old. Our sons Dennis and Michael were 13 and 16.

Dan was born and raised in Sudbury, Ontario the eldest son of Italian immigrants. He had a happy childhood, and was much loved and nourished by the fun-loving Italian community to which he belonged. He was good-looking and popular, did well in school, went on to university and graduated with a Bachelor of Mathematics, got married, had two sons, was very successful in his career, and had many friends. In short, he was living a charmed life.

Then he got cancer.
Life cracked open.

In the fall of 1992 Dan was diagnosed with rhabdomyosarcoma, a rare form of cancer that started in one of the large muscles of his right thigh. By the time the diagnosis was made, the cancer had already spread to the lymph nodes in his abdomen and to his lungs. Despite a poor prognosis, Dan agreed to embark on the most aggressive regimen of treatment available. This included chemotherapy, surgery, radiation, more chemotherapy, more radiation, a bone marrow transplant. He would do well, then he would do poorly. We would be optimistic, then our hopes would be shattered. By June 1994 it was clear that all medical avenues had been exhausted and the cancer was still progressing.

At the time he became ill, Dan was Assistant Vice-President of Marketing in the Individual Life Centre of Manulife, Canada's largest life insurance company. It was a job that required a high level of creative energy, something Dan had in abundance.

During the two years he was in active treatment Dan continued to work whenever he was able but there were periods when he was in hospital or was too sick or his blood counts were too low. His creative energy became refocused during these periods of forced stillness, taking him into previously unexplored parts of himself and the world around him.

Out of an increased need to express his feelings, Dan began to keep a personal journal in which he sketched, wrote poetry, recorded his thoughts and reflections. An extraordinary thing because he had never done any-thing like that before. Before his illness he rarely read unless it was work related, certainly did not read poetry; in fact he would have said that he did not like it, did not understand it.

As other new avenues of creativity opened up for him, he eagerly explored them all, delving deeper and deeper into himself and into his spiritual life. His creations, whether in clay, wood or words seemed to come out of his thirst to engage in the world despite his illness. This book, *Spiritual Warrior,* is Dan's expression of how he chose to engage in the world even as he prepared to leave it. It is the story of someone with an extraordinary will to live and to die with awareness, curiosity, faith and love.   It is not about life lived without pain, anxiety, anger and despair but about three years of Dan's life lived in the heightened awareness of all it means to be human.

Life cracked open.
The light got in.
Sometimes cancer does that.

Judy Blasutti

INTRODUCTION

In putting together *Spiritual Warrior* I found myself repeatedly bumping up against the same dilemma, that is how to maintain the integrity of Dan's work on the one hand and on the other how to deliver into the public domain a finished product that tells his story in a coherent fashion. During his illness Dan was writing a private journal, not a book. Because of this there are gaps, pieces missing, thoughts that seem to come out of nowhere, potential problems for a reader unfamiliar with Dan's illness and life.

A journalist friend, whom I asked to read Dan's journal, commented that no one gets to publish a book without an editor. As painful as it sometimes is to the ego of the writer, an editor is necessary, she says. But he's dead, I say. Somehow it seems unfair to tinker with his commas when he cannot defend them. Perhaps that comma has some cosmic significance! Eventually the absurdity of my thinking dawned on me: Dan no longer has an ego to wound. Further, he had himself thought of offering his journal to HopeSpring Cancer Support Centre as a fundraiser and had planned to review it before he died in order to fill in some of the gaps. He ran out of time.

Spiritual Warrior, therefore, does contain some editorial intervention where deemed necessary for clarity. This takes the form of footnotes in italics throughout the text. The journal itself remains very much as Dan wrote it. Entries are in chronological order with the date of each piece preceding it.

It was an editorial decision to divide the book into four sections in order to make it more reader-friendly. The breaks, however, are not arbitrary. There are definite shifts in Dan's work in terms of style, the kinds of issues he was exploring and where he was emotionally and spiritually.

The names of cancer patients Dan talks about in his journal have been changed to protect their privacy. Others whom he mentions – friends, family, and colleagues – have given permission for their names to be published.

His hope and mine is that *Spiritual Warrior* will be of help to others, in particular to those living with a life-threatening disease. Being confronted so directly with his mortality was an "eye opener" for Dan, a crisis that profoundly changed how he lived his life. His journal reflects how he managed to find opportunity, growth, creativity, love and joy even as he lived with cancer. To others confronted by a possibly fatal disease, this may offer a measure of hope and inspiration.

The book's broader appeal is to anyone on a journey of self-discovery and spiritual growth as Dan was.

Proceeds from the sale of this book will go to HopeSpring Cancer Support Centre with a portion being allocated to the *Spiritual Warrior Scholarship Fund*. This fund has been created in Dan's memory to provide educational assistance to young people whose lives have been touched by cancer. *The Spiritual Warrior Scholarship Fund* recognizes young individuals who most exemplify the characteristics exhibited by Dan. Dan was one of the founding members of HopeSpring and was a member of the Board when he died. HopeSpring is a non-residential centre for people living with cancer as well as their family and friends. The focus of programs at HopeSpring is to provide people with a variety of tools and techniques to help them cope with the stress of living with cancer or supporting someone with the disease.

Dan had been an Assistant Vice-President of Marketing in the Life Products division of Manulife Financial's Canadian Operations. During the three years he was ill, he maintained close ties with many of his colleagues and continued to work when he was able. He would have been pleased that the publication of *Spiritual Warrior* has been made possible by the generous financial support of his employer, Manulife Financial.

Judy Blasutti

I.

Eye Opener

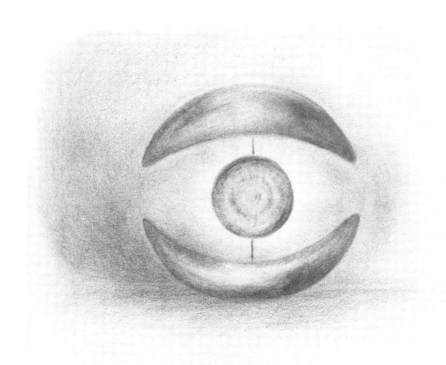

Victoria Hospital, London, Ontario
Here for my first chemotherapy treatment*
November 27, 1992

Eye Opener

I am so aware.
Colours are so bright.

I blink to ensure that they are real.
There are some I can actually feel.

I am so aware.
Emotions are so strong.
Wild happiness explodes from a child's smile,
Then fear attacks like a lurking crocodile.

I am so aware.
Love runs so deep.
I feel love all around me, everywhere.
My strength and courage stem from people who care.

I am so aware.

* Chemotherapy - the use of drugs to destroy cancer cells.
Chemotherapy drugs are usually given orally (by mouth) or intravenously (into a vein).

3

Until You're There

You don't realize you're there,
until you're there.
DETOUR
Where?

On the other side of your mind,
Now that's a find.
Why?

New thoughts, patterns, emotions,
A tremendous commotion.
What?

Well, it's almost out of control,
Yet a part of your soul.
How?

I don't know, don't ask me.
Take a peek and see.
Who?
You.

I am going back to the Detour.
Why?
'Cause I got nervous.

You hear the diagnosis.
You say "Yes" and gather courage,
And then three days of chemo,
It hits you like a ton of bricks.

Kitchener, Ontario
(Entries written in Kitchener are from home)
April 29, 1993

Oh Glorious River

Life's waters flow quickly, like a stream,
Babbling, gurgling, sparkling; a dream.
Occasionally resting peacefully in an eddy,
Then picking up
again, strong and steady.

What once was no more than a shining sliver,
Is now in full bloom a glorious river.
Forging her way through time, like forever,
Calling you to her side as passionate lover.

Dance with her aptly as she moves to and fro,
Hold on to her tightly, she's worth it you know.
Take each bend with lust and with zeal,
Open your heart to the beauty she'll reveal.

Kitchener, Ontario
At home recuperating from surgery to remove tumours
from leg and lymph nodes.
May 13, 1993

For You

It's for you I pray,
For whatever lies ahead
You can do it day by day,
Just like me in this bed.

It's for you I pray,
prayers to help you grow,
to help you find your way,
Oh how I love you so.

It's for you I pray,
So that you'll be strong,
And no matter what they say
Proudly sing your own song.

For you,
I pray.

Inside Out

Some say the cup's half empty,
Others protest it's half full.
Wrong.

The cup is overflowing,
And when yours does
You will know.

Inside out.

Paint,
Sculpt,
Write,
Sing,
Dance,
Plant,
Do your own thing.

Laugh,
Cry,
Explore,
Share,
Love,
Scream,
Listen, be aware.

Express yourself
and you'll find the pleasure of life.
And maybe you'll even find yourself.

The cup is not half empty,
The cup is not half full.
Right.
The cup is overflowing.

Victoria Hospital, London, Ontario
May 15, 1993

Visiting

We hide in the TV nook,
Obsessed in a best-selling book.
We hide behind the telephone
Easy escape to dial tone.

We hide behind "too busy man",
That works like a total ban.

I dream for "once upon a time",
A time much simpler than now.
I pray that we go full circle,
To a home much simpler than now.

Visit, you're welcome, drop by,
You don't need a reason why,
'Cause ever since the beginning,
People together meant singing.

It's just us, don't book an appointment
Bring yourself, we're our own entertainment.

I dream for "once upon a time",
A time much simpler than now.
I pray that we go full circle,
To a home much simpler than now.

Remember that we're just human,
We're child, man and woman,
Each has both good and bad
Sometimes ecstatic, sometimes mad.
And that's what's so interesting,
About people together visiting.

I dream for "once upon a time",
A time much simpler than now.
I pray that we go full circle,
To a home much simpler than now.

Victoria Hospital, London, Ontario
May 18, 1993

To My Special Friends

*(For my canoe buddies Mike Burke, John McEachen and Mark Shea)**

I want to be as good a friend,
As good to you
As you to me.
And how do I achieve this end?
The secret is in forever learning,
From what you say,
And what you do,
Through season after season turning.
As in old, a pledge of loyalty
Prick a finger,
Join the blood,
A bond more pure than royalty.
Then open up my heart to flower
I feel the warmth
The urge to grow
In your soothing light, protective tower.
Now...
No matter what the winds may send,
Through what I say,
And what I do
I want to be your faithful friend.
...Forever.

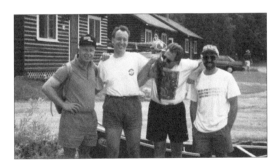

** Dan had a passionate affinity with nature and loved spending time outdoors. He had gone
on a wilderness canoe trip annually for eighteen years with his childhood friend, Mike Burke,
and another good friend, John McEachen, whom he met when he first started work after
graduating from university. Another friend, Mark Shea, whom Dan met while working at
Manulife, joined the trio about five years ago. These canoe trips and the friends he shared
them with were very important to Dan.*

Kitchener, Ontario
First night home after being five days in London for chemotherapy
May 18, 1993

Bedtime

I lie on my back,
Eyes closed,
And ask myself
To open.

I visualize
A red rose in full bloom,
Real close up.
And then a meadow,
And then a lake,
And then a sky,
And then the blinding
Sunlight,
Filling up to eternity.

I've opened.

Memories begin to swirl.
Excited eyes,
Rounding smiles,
Colourful laughter,
Favourite people,
Magic moments,
With champagne fizz.

Faded memories turn bright,
Life's new meanings are held in close,
It feels like heaven.

And then for some
Strange
Unknown reason,
I become reflective.
I turn onto my side
And pull up my legs,
I start to wonder.
I cry.
I grieve.
I die.

I wonder some more
About life,
About death,
About life again.
And I ask myself
To open up again.
Not as much as before
But I promise myself
That tomorrow,
I'll open up some more.

Kitchener, Ontario
May 23, 1993

Thought for the Day

I am experiencing an emotional freedom. I feel that I can express a greater range of emotions and to a much deeper level. Why? Foolishly perhaps, but I believe that others think this is expected or at least they find it tolerable because "he's got cancer, you know". What the hell, for whatever reason, I am allowing it to flow. While I hope to beat cancer and return to a "normal" life, I never want to return to my previous emotional life.

Life's Essence and Commitment

Think about it. You're seriously ill and lying in a hospital bed with loved ones around you. What do you have to give them? You can't run out and buy them a gift. You can't do something for them. What do you have left to give?

I think it boils down to this. You can give them love. Through your eyes, your smile, your touch and the expression of your thoughts and feelings you can both tell them and show them how much you love them.

And you can give them your example. You can show them that no matter what happens, life is worth living and that we all must have the hope and courage to carry on.

So now remove yourself from the constraints of illness and hospitals. Now what should you give? Give love. You have the freedom to give love in a million ways. And by leading through example you can prove, again in so many ways, that life is beautiful, that it's worth living. These are gifts worth giving. Committing yourself to giving them and then doing it is what life is really all about.

Kitchener, Ontario
May 28, 1993

A Tender Flame

There's a place I find where my mind looks back,
Where my heart starts racing, a train on a track,
And while it's a place I seldom go,
It's one I know is real and one I really know.

In the darkness I see a tender flame,
What glows inside is love in your name.
Dancing around in the flickering yellow and blue,
Are many memories of good times spent with you.

I've protected you from the erosive winds of time,
Fed you and fanned you, silent actor of mind,
And sure enough in a moment of need,
With soothing warmth you returned the deed.

It doesn't matter I don't see you anymore,
You're a part of my life I choose not to ignore.
I held you in the distant past,
And now I'm held by a flame meant to last.

To turn "A Tender Flame" (poem on page 14) into a country and western hurtin' song do as follows:

Verse 1   A minor / There's ....
                   F / Where .....
                   D minor / And ....
                   A minor / It's ....

Verse 2 is the chorus
                   C   / In .... G / a tender flame,
                   F   /What ....   C/ love   G/ in your name.
                   C   / Dancing ... G/ blue,
                   F   / Are... C/ times   G/ spent with you.

Verse 3 is the same as Verse 1
Verse 2 is the same as the chorus
Verse 4 is the same as Verse 1
Guitar picking on Verse 1 chords
Verse 2 is the same as the chorus
Repeat Verse 1
Verse 2 as chorus
Repeat chorus chord ending on 2 repeats of words, "a tender flame."

Kitchener, Ontario
Have been home a week from Manulife convention in Bermuda
June 11, 1993

Thank You Jack McFaull, Saskatoon

Because you were willing to share with me your experiences and methods, I've gained new insights into meditation, visualization and immunology. In fact, since our meeting I have been meditating, something I could not do before.

And I have never met so positive, active and young a person. Someone told me that you are in your 70s! My own standard for positiveness has moved up because of you and hopefully I'll achieve it.

Kitchener, Ontario
June 19, 1993

Ah-Ha!

All along I've been worried that I won't have the time to teach my kids ... and what to teach them and how to teach them etc. Of course the answer is right in front of my nose. Show them I love them.

Victoria Hospital, London, Ontario
Here for five-day chemo treatment
July 2, 1993

At a Coping with Cancer course that I attended on June 19th and 20th, I heard and learned many things that will be of value to me. One that sticks with me is the way one woman succinctly articulated one of the purposes of life. She advised that we first find our own uniqueness and then share this with the community. I like this approach.

Victoria Hospital, London, Ontario
July 4, 1993

It's amazing how powerful commonality is at opening friendship. Take Beth for instance, another cancer patient whom I met when I was in Victoria Hospital for chemotherapy. Her desire to talk to someone in a similiar situation is very high, as is mine. The warm-up period is very short and soon it seems that discussions can go to very deep levels. I find a sense of comfort and security in this. I see better now how group therapy can be so powerful a tool for healing.

Sharing on a personal level enhances the quality of life.

Victoria Hospital, London, Ontario
July 4, 1993

George has not been well on my last visits to him. He tires easily and his memory seems much worse. From time to time, he winces from pain due to the tumour on his brain.

I thank George for how he helped me when I was really down during my second 5-day chemo. Here was this 80 year-old marketing guy full of piss and vinegar. He noticed I was down and visited me regularly at my bedside to chat me up. I thought to myself that at 80 he's seen it all and is not afraid of death like me. WRONG! Late one evening I heard him speaking to a friend on the phone. He said, "I'm dying, don't you see that. I'm dying and I don't want to die." Boy that took me by surprise, and I really don't know why when I look back. Age is not chronological. Readiness for death is not age specific. Youth is defined by the heart. George, by every standard, is young at heart. So am I. That's why we don't want to die yet. We love life.

Thank you George for your support in my time of need. I hope that I can do the same for you.

Victoria Hospital, London, Ontario
July 21, 1993

Thoughts About Louisa

In so short a time we developed an interesting friendship of mutual support. You give me those compliments which make me smile and feel like a kid. I give you a moment of undivided attention which seems to relieve your loneliness. You say that you've never seen such bright eyes and enthusiastic smile. Well, your eyes are incredibly full of sparkle and youth and your smile has a twist of mischievousness.

I was surprised at the happiness you expressed when the doctors said you had only nine months to live. I told you not to listen to the doctors, that you should decide to live longer. But you said that you were ready. That you believed your favourite people (father, mother, husband, sister, and many close friends) were in heaven and that you'd join them. What more could you ask for although you say that you would miss your four boys and grandchildren because you love them very much.

I was angry, sad and generally confused by your attitude. It has taken me weeks to understand it. I was imposing my own feelings and attitudes on you. All my favourite people are here on earth. I've not lost one, ever. I don't want to die because I want to be here with them. Your beliefs mean that you escape loneliness to join your loved ones. I fear leaving everyone and being alone. At times I have thought patterns and emotions that overcome this fear. Or I read or hear something that gives me courage. But I still basically fear death and do not want to die — at least not yet.

Having thought about your situation, I have been trying to put myself in your shoes, age 75 with what seems to have been a very full and active life. Now your illness has confined you in many ways and you feel lonely. I can rationalize your point of view and maybe I can even understand it a bit.

Louisa, I look forward to seeing you again and in the meantime I'll pray that you get what you want.

Kitchener, Ontario
August 1993

In The Middle

It feels like such a long time.
Eight months of treatment so far
and another six damn treatments to go.
I still get angry at this injustice
and want so badly for it all to end.

It is so much an uncertain time.
The only thing I know for sure
Is another radiation blast tomorrow.
I've heard the odds; but I'm different
I have to hope that I'll be one to mend.

Oh, I worry that there may be too little time;
I've met people who lived only a few months
and others who lived many years, you know.
I have a sense of urgency to get things done,
to spend time with both family and friends.

Yes, life does go on in the meantime;
growing boys have birthdays and parties.
There are at least a thousand ideas to sow.
Relationships change with each new struggle
But it's the consistency of love that I want to send.

I do try to live it "one day at a time",
Live the moment, keep my sight on the horizon.
I wish that I really learned this long ago.
I enjoy this approach to overcoming my fears,
For healing inside and out are just as important in the end.

Victoria Hospital, London, Ontario
August 29, 1993

The Rose Garden at "Hotel Vic" * is my favourite place to go now that
I'm mobile enough to make it here with IV pole and all. I roll my IV pole
under an old oak tree, take off my shoes, sit down and immediately relax.
On weekdays there is a constant chatter of children at play across the yard
in a Hospital Day Care Centre. In this place, with feet grounded in the
grass, I am able to meditate and do relaxation exercises easily. I wish
more patients could get out of their rooms to enjoy this.

* *"Hotel Vic" was Dan's nickname for Victoria Hospital in London, Ontario where
he had most of his cancer treatments.*

Kitchener, Ontario
September 20, 1993

Thought For The Day

> Everything can be taken from a man but one thing: the last of
> the human freedoms - to choose one's attitude in any given set
> of circumstances, to choose one's own way.[2]
> -Victor E. Frankl, *Man's Search for Meaning*

In my own search for meaning over the last nine months, I have often
thought about attitude and my ability to choose and maintain a positive
attitude regardless of the circumstances. I read the above quote in Bernie
Siegel's* new book *Peace, Love and Healing*[3] just at a time when I needed
to be reminded that I am in control of my attitude.

* *Bernie S. Siegel, M.D. is the author of several books dealing with living with cancer.
Dr. Siegel's approach is to promote greater awareness of the mind/body connection.
Dan found his books very inspiring.*

Kitchener, Ontario
September 30, 1993

"Garbage Out" For The Day

I've been back at work now for most of this month. I must admit that I do find my work intellectually stimulating and that I have fun while I'm there. However, I have moments of frustration as well because I value my time so greatly and can't stand any bit of it being wasted.

I find that I am exhausted by five o'clock and have little energy for other things. I must recognize this as a sign and not push myself until I find my energy levels are completely back.

Victoria Hospital, London, Ontario
Here for a five-day chemo
October 22, 1993

Mind Body/Body Mind

I was quite impressed by Deepak Chopra's* lecture on Monday night in London and have started reading his book *Quantum Healing*.[4] The basic premise is that the mind is not a subset of the body; instead the body is a subset of the mind. This is a completely new paradigm and the new thoughts and ideas emanating from this approach are very stimulating. Is there really a mind/body connectiveness and thus a mind/body approach to medicine and healing? I am absolutely convinced that there is.

I intend to explore and learn further in this area and hope to gain further insights into healing and spirituality.

---

* *Deepak Chopra, M.D. was born and raised in New Delhi, India and is a pioneer in the West on the subject of mind/body medicine. He taught at Tufts University and Boston University Schools of Medicine and became chief of staff at New England Memorial Hospital. He established the American Association of Ayurvedic Medicine, bringing together his own interest and knowledge of Eastern medical practice with medical practice in the West. He has authored many successful books and has had his work translated into more than twenty-five languages.*

Transcendental Meditation

After a few attempts at meditating based on "how to" books, I was finally motivated to get trained in transcendental meditation. The result was excellent. I've been meditating for nine days now, twice a day, and find that I have more energy during the day and have been sleeping better as well.

The motivation for TM training came in part from listening to Dr. Chopra at a seminar in London. I bought two of his books and as a result have gone to an Ayurvedic* doctor for an assessment. I have learned that I am Pitta-Kapha body type and the doctor prescribed a number of teas and herbs. I haven't decided if I should follow this yet.

* *The term ayurveda is derived from two Sanskrit words: "Ayus" meaning life and "veda" meaning science or knowledge. This "science of life" is generally considered to be India's traditional medicine. It is a practice of medicine that has a deep spiritual basis . Ayurvedic medicine has identified three body types, namely vata, pitta, and kapha, each of which has its own needs, strengths and vulnerabilities.*

University Hospital, London, Ontario
November 9, 1993

Magnetic Resonance Imagery (MRI)

This will be the third MRI* and probably the one I am most anxious about. The first confirmed my diagnosis. The second was a check point on progress. This is now the one to see if the chemo, surgery, and radiation have done the job. I suspect that they'll find a lot of damage from the chemo and radiation. I really hope that they don't find any remaining tumours. Now that I'm back to work and things seem to be normal, I am wanting this to continue.

I'm getting excited about work. I have established a good balance of doing things for myself, work and family time.

A good MRI and CATSCAN* offers so much hope. If it's not, then I'll have to continue to fight and try not to give up hope.

MRI and CATSCAN are two highly sophisticated diagnostic tools used to produce detailed images or pictures of a specific area of the body. These images are then studied and interpreted by a radiologist who reports the findings to other physicians involved in the case.

Owen Sound, Ontario
Visiting my brother-in-law and his family
(Judy's brother Frank is a radiologist)
November 26, 1993

Phew!

Good news. All tumour sites seem to be free of tumours now. The MRI of the leg was good. Frank reviewed the CATSCAN of the abdomen and says it looks good. He also received the year's history of lung X-rays and feels that the lungs are also tumour free.

Yesterday marked the one year anniversary of the first chemo treatment. Man, I've come a long way! The first poem in this book was written one year ago tomorrow.

The intensity of my awareness has decreased a little but is still far above what was normal for me before my diagnosis. While I am optimistic, there is still uncertainty, actually a great deal of uncertainty, about the future, therefore I look to maximize every day.

I can clearly remember my first five-day chemo treatment. I was scared. I cried often. One of my favourite nurses hugged me and consoled me. A patient next door to me, a woman who had suffered a number of recurrences, heard me crying one day and stopped by my room to talk to me and offer me hope. Judy spent a lot of time with me, encouraging me to fight even though she was as terrified as I was.

Over the last year I have had tremendous support from so many people. It's incredible. My family has been there consistently. My friends, old and new, have been so helpful.

Thanks for a great year!

II.

Hope

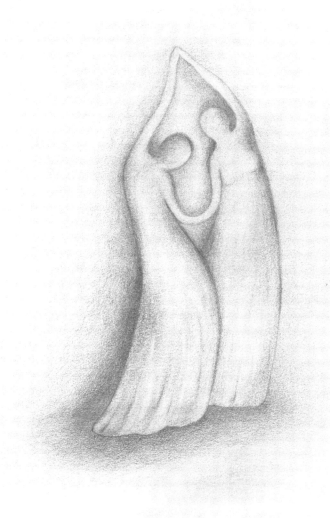

Victoria Hospital, London, Ontario
December 13, 1993

Spring Will Come

When winter's howling wind
Gnashes at the darkest hour,
I relive a moment.
A bright spring day.
The dancing breeze.
Its silky touch,
On yearning skin.
Rejuvenating.
Hope.

Kitchener, Ontario
December 19, 1993

Midnight Dance

As I lie here
Listening to soft music
I long for a mere
Trace of your familiar scent,
And your warmth near
Enough to touch and hold.

As you lie there,
Reading another poetry book,
As one of a pair
Do you look up to sense me,
Suspended in the air
With arms inviting you up?

Come together
In our imagination,
Light as a feather
We'll dance to our own song,
One together
Entwined in life's mystery.

As I lie here
Lost in this heartbreaking dance,
A loosened tear
Runs down my dry-skinned cheek,
For you, my dear.
Love runs very, very deep.

Kitchener, Ontario
January 14, 1994

Happy New Year!

This is the first day this year that I've felt like writing and the first day that I am happy for the New Year. Until now I've been mainly angry and anxious. Angry for a whole pile of reasons including wishing this thing was all over. Anxious because of all the waiting for and qualifying for the bone marrow transplant.

But today I feel much better. Yesterday I had my last chemo of the fifteen-course treatment. Since November 15, 1992 I've gone through fifteen chemos, one surgery and thirty-three radiation* blasts! Over the next two weeks, I will have an MRI (today) and CATSCANs of my belly and chest. If all goes well, later in February I get a bone marrow test. If my bone marrow is cancer-free and I stay healthy (underlined as a reminder to myself to not get sick), then it's all systems go in March or April for the Bone Marrow/Chemo procedure.*

I had a session with my therapist today and found it very useful and, as usual, he was very supportive.

I'm looking forward to Arizona in terms of doing business, seeing the managers and spending a few days of holidays with Judy.

Radiation Therapy - the use of particles or waves to destroy cancer cells.

Bone Marrow/Chemo Procedure - Dan did have this procedure in March 1994. It is sometimes called an analogous bone marrow transplant (because no donor is involved) or a bone marrow rescue.

This procedure involves the re-injection of previously extracted bone marrow cells after extremely high doses of chemotherapy. Bone marrow is contained in the centre of the bone where all blood cells (red cells, white cells and platelets) are formed. Red cells carry oxygen, white cells fight infection and platelets prevent bleeding.

Before high-dose chemotherapy could safely be given to Dan, healthy bone marrow cells were extracted from his hip and stored as liquid until needed later. High-dose chemotherapy was given in an attempt to eradicate any remaining cancer cells. In the process, bone marrow cells were also damaged, putting Dan at risk of hemorrhaging or contracting a fatal infection. This is where the transplant comes in. The stored healthy cells were given back to Dan through his Hickman intravenous line. These cells found their way back into the bone marrow and were able to start producing healthy blood cells again.

31

Kitchener, Ontario
January 15, 1994

Little Koala Bear
(for my friend Carrie Parker*)

There sits a little koala
Beside my bed,
He's always looking at me
With a turned head,
And in this way reminds me
Of what you said,
Yes, such a little gesture
And so much said.

* *Carrie is a wonderful friend who worked with Dan at Manulife. One time before Dan was going into hospital, Carrie came by with a little stuffed Koala Bear that she had bought in Australia and which she had carried with her for good luck for many years. She wanted Dan to take a memento of her caring and friendship with him into hospital.*

Victoria Hospital, London, Ontario
February 28, 1994

(This was the first day of what would be a 33-day stay in hospital for high doses of chemotherapy and a bone marrow "rescue" procedure. Dan had anticipated being in hospital for six to eight weeks but his recovery went more quickly.)

The test results came in...leg OK, abdomen OK, lungs problematic. The cancer is already coming back. Man, am I pissed off!

Today, while I wait for a bone marrow harvest, I'm less angry and much more worried. Knowing that the next six to eight weeks will be rough, I can't help wondering if it will be worth it. On the other hand, it is a glimmer of hope, hope for a remission and maybe a cure.

I'll have to keep my eye on the horizon while I ride out the storm... and I can feel a storm brewing.

Victoria Hospital, London, Ontario
March 2, 1994

The bone marrow extract went well and I recovered quickly although I still have aches and pains.

Today at South Street Campus, I had a Hickman Line* put in by a very friendly and professional staff. The line was in and in no time at all. During the procedure one of the nurses chatted me up and kept me relaxed and after I managed to bum 75 cents from her for a coffee!

My isolation room for the bone marrow transplant is looking good. I have a CD player, VCR/TV, computer hooked into work, a stationary bike and lots of books. I think I'll be able to keep myself busy and up for the whole stay.

---

* Hickman Line - an intravenous tube that is surgically implanted into a major blood vessel close to the heart. It is used to administer chemotherapy, blood products and bone marrow.

Victoria Hospital, London, Ontario
March 2, 1994

Hold On

Touch me,
Hold on to my hand.

Love me,
Hold on to my heart.

Victoria Hospital, London, Ontario
March 3, 1994

Kneel Down

In order to heal,
I think I must peel
Away the layers of costumes,
Strip off all of my purchased clothes.

In order to heal,
I think I must feel
Well beyond my fabled roles
And connect with the ebbs and flows.

In order to heal,
I think I must kneel,
And only then, can I stand up
Holding the glorious red rose.

Victoria Hospital, London, Ontario
March 12, 1994

While covering up the IV pump with a blanket the other night, I recalled how I used to cover up the canary at night when I was a kid. I told this to a nurse while getting a back rub and she told me similar childhood stories. As I lay there, I remembered how my mother would talk of her father and his large walk-in cage full of the canaries that he raised. It was a good feeling, being mothered and being emotionally connected to the past.

Victoria Hospital, London, Ontario
March 18, 1994

Judy told me that Mike woke up in the middle of the night calling "Daddy, Daddy, Daddy." God, that hurts.

Victoria Hospital, London, Ontario
March 21, 1994

Hush Now

"Daddy, Daddy, Daddy."

Gone. Nowhere. Not to be found,
In a dream hitting the ground.
Found only in a boy's heart
Where he has been from the start.

Hush now, do not be afraid.
What else is there to be said?

Oh God, so big is this heart
Head hung low, kick in the dirt.
Such a giant cross to bear
Shoulders, please be strong and square.

Oh how much love for the child.
It hurts. Emotions run wild.

"Daddy, Daddy, Daddy."
Hush now, do not be afraid.
I love you.

Hush now.

Victoria Hospital, London, Ontario
March 27, 1994

Well, this is the 28th day in the Hotel Vic, the 18th in isolation. I think I have done well so far. This morning I called Judy. I was a bit down and bored but I pulled myself out of it within an hour.

My white blood cell count continues to fluctuate and this is what's so frustrating. Things in my control are going really well. Blood counts are out of my control; I can't seem to tell them what to do. I have to remember that I've had lots of chemo over the last 16 months and a very high dose only three weeks ago.

Had a great evening singing away to love songs by different artists on CDs at volume level eight. Some of the nurses hung out in the meds room again singing with me!

Victoria Hospital, London, Ontario
March 30, 1994

21st Day of Isolation/31 Days in Hotel Vic

I jested with Judy today that I couldn't leave the Hotel Vic unless I got to bring my "red" button home with me.

The red button is tied to my bed and calls the nursing station. They answer "Hi Dan, how can I help?" to which I respond "Nurse please" or "Could someone send in a popsicle please." They say that it takes 30 days to develop a habit. Well in these last thirty days I developed a little habit - the little red button, my security blanket. I guess it'll be "cold turkey" when I get home!

Victoria Hospital, London, Ontario
March 31, 1994

Well, I must admit that I really did prepare myself well for this last month, especially in terms of having things to keep me busy. The computer link to work has been a great source of communication with people at Manulife and I kept up-to-date as a side benefit. The TV/VCR from Leo and the CD player from Dennis both turned out great as Judy, the nurses, and even another patient's husband brought in CDs and tapes regularly. I've taped about fifteen 100-minute audio tapes.

Following a daily schedule and doing meditations also helps tremendously. Often a nurse drops in before shift or during break to spend 10 or 15 minutes to chat - I really appreciate this. Judy visits every other day and still runs the homestead and keeps As in her courses. Family calls daily to chat and friends regularly. I have tons of support.

Sometime in April I'll be out of here and I am a bit anxious about it because it'll mean coming back to London Regional Cancer Centre for tests and results. Sure hope this worked.

Kitchener, Ontario
May 6, 1994

Test results are encouraging but not conclusive. It'll be two or three months before we know more. More waiting — more living with uncertainty.

Dad's minor heart attack and the discovery of an aneurism on his abdominal aeorta was not the greatest news. On the other hand, finding out now before something major happened to him is probably a blessing. We'll have to wait to see what the heart tests show.

Back at work and I think it will be fun. I look forward to the marketing services assignment that I'll be doing.

I haven't really felt myself and I'm not sure why. I can't seem to meditate well these days and for the last week I've almost lost the habit. I seem to have lost my creativity, high energy level and high motivation level. I can honestly say I don't like myself like this. Part of the reason I'm sure are the things Judy and I are going through right now. Hopefully I'll work myself out of it soon.

Kitchener, Ontario
June 14, 1994

It's been a while since I have written in my journal. I think a major reason is that with full-time work I am very tired at the end of the day. I've not done anything creative since my return to work. However, at work I feel that I am contributing and creative so that's where my energy is going.

Overall, things are going quite well. Judy and I are getting along; the kids are busy with baseball and other things.

I am a bit anxious about going to London on Thursday because I may get some news. A CATSCAN is scheduled for early July — so July will bring more news.

Prince Edward Island
July 3, 1994

I am now sipping coffee in a cottage near Chelton Beach, P.E.I.!*

On June 16th, I received news that the bone marrow transplant was not successful in that a few remaining spots (i.e. tumours) were still on the lungs. My oncologist was clear on the point that the cancer could come back quickly and that options are limited. However, I am pushing her to explore all the options and I am going to review alternative treatments and therapies myself.

After a fantastic canoe trip down the French River, I told my family and the people at work about the tumours in my lungs. I decided to take long-term disability as of July 1st so that I'll have time off to do things with my family. As Mom and Dad were joining my brother Robert, his wife Debbie and family in P.E.I. for a week, we decided to join them.

The first night of the trip was in Montreal where Dale Congram *(Manulife Branch Manager)* and his family took us out for dinner in the old town. We had a great time. The second night was in Grand Falls, New Brunswick where we met up with the family. Yesterday we had brunch in Fredricton and arrived here in P.E.I. for supper. I'm looking forward to a fun week.

When I get back, I'll focus on what to do about the cancer.

* With the news that the bone marrow transplant was unsuccessful and the cancer back in his lungs, Dan realized his prognosis was not good. He asked his oncologist how long she predicted he might live. Although she was unable to be certain, she said he wouldn't likely survive a year. Thinking this might be his last summer, Dan wanted to spend time with his family, to travel, to enjoy life while he still felt well. We vacationed on Canada's East Coast in July and West Coast in August. It was an action-packed summer! Very enjoyable.

Kitchener, Ontario
July 15, 1994

Boy, yesterday was a tough day with news that the cancer is in both lungs and growing at a moderate pace. The conventional options do not look promising. It was very tough breaking the news to family. There are going to be some very hard and sad days ahead so I'd better make the most of the good ones now.

Today was a fantastic day at Manulife as I was given special recognition for my volunteer work with the Cancer Society.* A ton of people showed up and many nice things were said. I was truly flattered by the personal donations of $3,000 that people made in honour of my special recognition.

* *Dan had been chair of the business fundraising campaign for the Canadian Cancer Society. He developed a marketing plan for increasing corporate donations and had recruited a team of volunteers to carry out the plan.*

Kitchener, Ontario
July 22, 1994

Yesterday I gave a 30-minute speech to Manulife's Hamilton Branch.*
I thought it went well. I could sense the attentiveness of the audience and
could hear a pin drop. Rod, the Branch Manager, wrote me saying it was
perfect and that many had mentioned to him that they were close to tears.
This confirms what I felt in the room. I was worried that it was a bit
heavy but then again heavy is also a part of life.

I really enjoyed my sister Marilyn's visit this week. While we didn't
get into any major discussions, her presence was comforting to me.

My visit with my therapist went well. I was struggling with a fear — a
fear of giving up. I feel like I am accepting the situation fully but my fear
lies in this — If I have accepted this, does it mean I've given up? We dis-
cussed this at length after which I concluded that acceptance and giving up
were not at all the same. The key still remains to live each day to the
fullest.

Went to a naturopath for my first consultation. She said that I'd have
to make a lot of changes to my diet in particular. Things like coffee and
cheese would have to go! I have a week or so to think about what I will
decide.

* *Although Dan had taken long-term disability and was no longer working at Manulife on a
regular basis, he would sometimes be invited to speak at a branch meeting. He enjoyed this
as a way to keep in contact with many of the Manulife people he had worked with over the
years. He felt a great deal of support and caring from his Manulife colleagues.*

Vancouver, British Columbia
On holidays with Judy, Dennis and Mike
August 6, 1994

Vancouver —- what a great city! So far we are having fun although we are all suffering from jet lag.

Yesterday we went to the top of Grouse Mountain. I really enjoyed the view and the time we spent hiking around. A moment that I will remember is when I meditated for ten minutes on top of the mountain. I sat on an old log which was about four feet wide (I had to jump up onto it) and gained a tremendous feeling of serenity, a sense of timelessness.

Vancouver Island
August 10, 1994

We are having a fantastic time here at Tofino in Clayoquot Sound on Vancouver Island. We've hiked in the rainforest, along Long Beach and best of all, yesterday we went on a seven-hour boat trip. The first two hours on the way to Hot Springs Cove, we saw sea lions, grey whales, a porpoise and countless birds, including bald eagles. We then stopped and hiked 30 minutes through an old-growth forest to the hot springs. This was a real blast and according to our guide the temperature of the water is 43 degrees Celcius!

After hiking back to the boat we came back through the inland waterway and saw black bears on the beach. The sunset was magnificent. One can easily see how the artists in this area are inspired and why they use such reds and purples in their paintings.

This morning the tide was out as I walked along the beach. Very peaceful. Very beautiful.

L'Chaim

"L'chaim." Yiddish for "To Life." I learned this from a most interesting older Jewish man, Morris Raizman, who is an agent in the Winnipeg East Branch. He was a Maldanek Camp survivor and spent six years in concentration camps in his late teens and early 20s. He spoke many languages, including fluent Italian. He claims that he was really born in Rome because it was in Rome after he was liberated from the camps by the Red Army that he first knew freedom. We had some interesting chats which I really enjoyed.

I had a good time at the Winnipeg East branch getaway at Gunn Lake. Glen McHugh and Pat Gill were very interesting speakers and I picked up many good ideas.

The fishing was a blast as we caught many pickerel and other fish.

I felt very confident as I told my story today. I talked for over an hour and my delivery was strong. The response I received was tremendous. I hit the emotional heart of everyone in the room and many were in tears. Many people came up after the meeting to thank me and give me a hug. A few came up to me at lunch still with tears in their eyes and thanked me for a moving and inspirational talk. All wished me well in my future. This has been very gratifying.

"L'chaim."

Kitchener, Ontario
September 8, 1994

The last week and a half was a tough one. I have been experiencing severe pain in my back and after a few days of trying to treat it as a back problem, I went to the doctor. Seems that the tumours on the lower lobe of my left lung caused an inflamation internally (on the pleural lining) which caused pain where the lining attaches to the shoulder and back. This certainly brought home the reality of my disease, especially since I've felt so good all summer. I had a chat with my sons, Dennis and Michael, which was very hard on me emotionally. Who knows how fast the disease will progress? But I feel as ready as one can be to handle it.

Kitchener, Ontario
September 8, 1994

Listen

Sit still.
Listen.
What do I hear?

Within the hypnotic beat of life
The constant ring of silence,
And there, timeless memory
Flows in a continuous stream.

Above the persistent sound of drums
The shamans cry healing chants;
This powerful poetry
Initiates vision through a dream.

From the full and rhythmic dance of love
The breathtaking joy of life
And peaceful serenity
Completes life's neverending theme.

Kitchener, Ontario
October 15, 1994

It's been a long time since I've written.   September was a hard month
of physical pain. October has been back and forth to London for radiation.
I've been generally sad although I have had some bright moments.
The operations that Dad has gone through have also taken an emotional
toll and seeing him in hospital has been tough on me.

Kitchener, Ontario
October 15, 1994

It's not like surrendering to the light. It becomes a desire to go freely,
knowing that after the final anguish, Rebirth.

Kitchener, Ontario
October 31, 1994

The last two weeks I've been very tired from the radiation. I do see improvement each day but I am not feeling myself yet.

The week in Sudbury was spent between the hospital and my parent's place. Dad was very ill and weak while I was there. I felt that I was helpful and supportive for Mom and Marilyn and I feel good about that.

After a week of deliberating how much time I can give to the Cancer Society, I decided that I must be firm and let them know (again) that they must find a replacement. This was difficult for me but it is the best solution for them and me.

Kitchener, Ontario
November 17, 1994

I've been back into radiation again since Monday, November 14th. Today, before my radiation appointment, I met with a nurse who asked me if I was still writing poetry. I had to confess that I had fallen out of the habit of writing at all. I used to carry this book in my knapsack all the time up until September and it's time for it to go back in.

The first round of radiation was very effective and I've not felt pain or needed morphine since. After much deliberation I decided to go ahead with the second round. Part of the reason is that the tumour growth on the lungs has stabilized. The more important part is that I value walking so much that I'll put up with another two weeks of treatments and another three to four weeks to feel better. Here's hoping these treatments are effective and long-lasting.

I'm also taking a host of naturopathic medicines from my naturopath. She is also giving me a weekly Integrated Touch session for free. She certainly has a strong healing presence and a very caring attitude.

Dad is finally off dialysis and, while he is weak due to low blood counts, I'm certain he'll be fully recovered in another month or so.

Kitchener, Ontario
November 20, 1994

Creativity

I was reading the Nov/Dec '94 issue of *Sculpture* magazine and was fascinated by the interview with Donald Saff who is an artist/educator. When asked, "Have you come to a conclusion that art-making is an in-born predilection?" he responded at length.

Here's the first part of his response: "No, I have not come to that conclusion. I've come to the conclusion that I have no ability to speculate on the best way to predict or educate an artist. Or the best way to evaluate art, for that matter. Effective education depends on the construct of the individual. Some people bloom early, others late. Insight and urge to express is a time variable."[5]

I like his approach and particularly agree with the last line. The "time variable" for me has been my illness and desire to express feelings or concepts that are swirling around in me. I also like the idea that he hints at, the point that we all have creative or artistic talents.

This is supported by Tom Harpur in his book *God Help Us*[6]. In his article titled "The Creative Spirit" Harpur states that as we are "like God" we have the "power to choose, to make moral decisions; it means having the capacity for self-reflective thought; above all, it means the gift of creativity". Later in the article, he states that in order to find your uniqueness and originality you must be "fully yourself. Since each of us is unique, the reality we know and express will inevitably have its own unique quality or slant." Besides listening in solitude to yourself, he prescribes acquiring "the habit of eccentricity" and learning "to think holistically."

Now with this as background, I'd like to reflect on my own situation and artistic growth. I started complaining of illness in May '92. That summer we went to Italy, where I was awestruck by all the art, especially the magnificent sculpture. Over a two-year period, prior to going to Italy, I was building a wood carving tool collection with some vague notion that I wanted to start sculpting more. While in Italy, this notion became a vision. I could see myself as an old person working on sculptures.

After the shock of diagnosis, which forced me into a new perspective, I was influenced by Bernie Siegel's books to do goal setting. Three of my goals are to increase my spirituality, to express my emotions in a variety of ways (talking, writing, painting, sculpture, etc.) and to become a master sculptor by my old age. The last goal was and is a way of keeping the long term healing view alive.

Another point that I'd like to add to Harpur's formula is that you must let go of fear - fear of what others might think about your work - otherwise you'll be paralyzed in action. It's better to just do it. That doesn't mean you can't ask for input/discussion/help on your ideas.

With all this in mind, I started out on my journey.

There is a spiritual dimension to the work I've done over the last two years. And as I was reviewing my work this morning, I had an idea I'm excited about. I intend to explain some of my work so as to capture the emotions and the thoughts I was feeling, again as a way to continue to express myself fully.

Descriptions of Some of My Sculptures

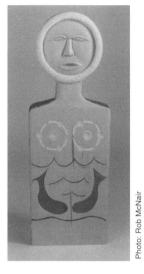

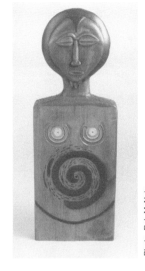

Photo: Rob McNair

Photo: Rob McNair

TWO FACES, ONE QUEST - 1993 - Wood, acrylic paints (34" high)
There are many unconscious spiritual symbols in this work. In this and other pieces, I am impacted by the anima perspective that Carl Jung talks about.

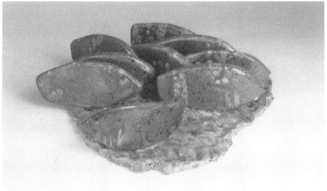

Photo: Rob McNair

INDIVIDUALITY - 1994 - Clay (4" high x 15" wide)
Eight fish swim in one direction while a more colourful one swims away. The title evokes a thought that this one fish is bold enough to be different. At a much deeper level, the colourful fish is nearing death. Two colour changes are significant: the blue of the ocean (the fish's universe) has appeared in the one fish's eye and mid-body (heart), and a bit of raw clay is exposed (flesh) all symbolizing a spiritual growth toward being with the universe and God.

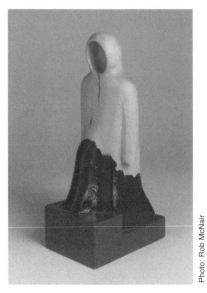

OUT OF THE MUD - 1993
Basswood (10" high)
One must go through the mud (the suffering in life) in order to climb the stairs to God.

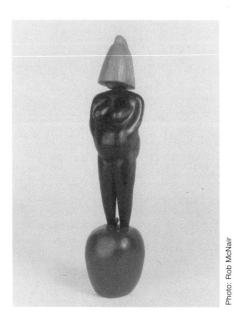

GREAT MOTHER EARTH FERTILITY GODDESS - 1993- Basswood (14" high)
Inspired by the Clan of the Cavebear series by Jean Auel. Subconsciously, I implanted her into an apple to represent the harvest and inadvertently connected her to Eve.

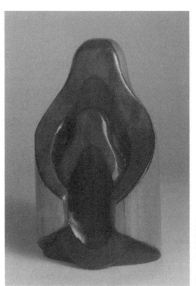

CARING - 1993 - Basswood (9" high)
This represents caring for the child within, where the spiritual light resides.

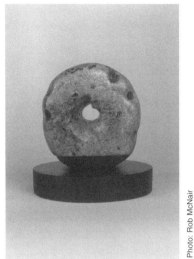

MUSIC - 1993 - Soapstone (7" high)
This is an attempt at abstract. It's representative of a whole note, an ear, a musical instrument. I intend it to evoke the wholeness and harmony that is present in nature.

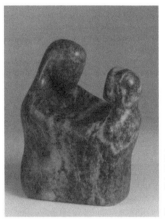

MOTHER AND 7 YEAR-OLD CHILD - 1992
Soapstone (7" high)
Inspired by the hundreds of mother and child sculptures and paintings I saw in Italy during the summer of '92. I wanted to capture the unique connectiveness between a mother and an older child rather than the babies and toddlers usually depicted.

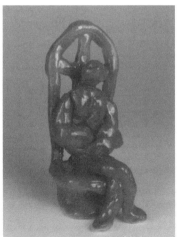

TWISTED - 1994 - Clay (9" high)
I was feeling depressed and in emotional knots when I twisted two ropes of clay into a human form with head hung low.

Kitchener, Ontario
December 19, 1994

Six days until Christmas. Physically I'm feeling well and count my blessings for this. However, I'm on Prednisone for a drug allergy to Naprosyn and I seem to be very moody the last few days. Anger that has built up in me is being unleashed on some poor unsuspecting souls like Judy, Dennis and Michael. I've been trying to let it go in meditation or yoga chants. While these techniques help temporarily, the littlest thing can set me off an hour later.

So what is the anger about? At the unfairness of it all. How it's played out these last few months. Exciting things are happening at work and I'm sitting on the sidelines. Yet these bursts of anger serve to push people away. I think I'm usually better able to control myself so I wonder if the Prednisone side effect of mood swings is complicating things. Nonetheless, I feel angry. My needs are not being met and I'll have to cope with it.

Kitchener, Ontario
January 8, 1995

Christmas was just what I needed. I really enjoyed Christmas Eve and morning at home with Judy, Dennis and Michael. Christmas at the farm was a great time and Christmas at home with Mom, Dad, Marilyn and Robert and his family was also a good time. During all of this I didn't have time to think of things that were making me angry and ever since, I've mellowed considerably.

Unfortunately, I ran into some physical issues after Christmas — hernia, flu, pluerisy-type pain and a bad rash. I coped through these (just barely) and now with the help of Prednisone the rash and lung pain are under control.

I saw my oncologist on January 5 and received disappointing news. Why I would expect anything else is beyond me, but I still hope for the best and for slow tumour growth. Since November a number of new tumours have appeared on my lungs. This news makes me question again everything that I am doing. I am getting more involved in work with the new marketing department and am really enjoying the mental stimulation. But it takes energy and time. When I ask myself what else I could be doing during the day when the kids and Judy are busy, most of the activities are creative or spiritual in nature. I am going to try to balance this over the next two or three weeks. I also need and want to save enough energy for the end of the day for family and friends but find this difficult because by 7 p.m. I'm tired out and by 9 p.m. I am needing to be in bed.

About mid-December I started yoga under Pat Carty's* instruction. I really have found this useful both from a physical and mental point of view. The stretching and breathing exercises are relaxing. The chanting is a good substitute for my transcendental meditation practice which I lost in the fall of '94 when I was on morphine.

Pat loaned me a couple of books which I found very useful: one on the power of the mantra and another on working with Light as a meditative force. I've always liked working with Light, right from when I was first introduced to it at the "Helping Yourself" course at Wellspring in Toronto in June '93. It comes naturally to me, so I think I'm going to incorporate Light into my daily routine.

Pat Carty has been encouraging me to journal regularly and to dump all my feelings into it, however I just don't feel comfortable with that process. At times I'd rather be firm and tough with negative feelings or thoughts as they arise by saying "STOP" or finding a diversion. The risk of course is that they bubble away under the surface. Oh well.

*Pat Carty is a certified yoga instructor in Kitchener. Along with Dan, she is one of the founders of HopeSpring. She became Dan's yoga teacher, friend and spiritual companion during the last year of his life.

Kitchener, Ontario
January 10, 1995

Over the past few days I've been reading a couple of books that Pat
Carty gave me on mantras and meditations. I've found these books very
useful and I particularly like the meditation practice called "The Divine
Light Invocation." I've done this for three days in a row and find it a very
spiritual and healing experience.

> I am created by Divine Light.
> I am sustained by Divine Light.
> I am protected by Divine Light.
> I am surrounded by Divine Light.
> I am ever growing into Divine Light.

> Every cell of this, my physical body, is filled with
> Divine Light. Every level of consciousness is illumined
> with Divine Light. The Divine Light penetrates every
> single cell of my being, every level of consciousness.
> I have become a channel of pure Light. I am one with
> the Light.[7]

> – Swami Sivananda Radha
> *The Divine Light Invocation*

Kitchener, Ontario
January 14, 1995

We received a letter from the widow of a patient, whom I'd met in London, who just recently died. He was a young guy just like me with a similar kind of cancer. This hit Judy pretty hard. It hit me too. Today I couldn't resist reading the letter again and the material sent about the funeral. One piece was written by Brad in September '94 about his spiritual house. I was very touched by this, especially the part about unfinished rooms that included one for his family. While I haven't carried anger as long as Brad did, I have felt its depth. Right now I don't carry anger but I do feel a great sadness about the pain and suffering that Judy, Dennis, Michael and my family will feel in the future. I feel at a loss about what to do for them or how to prepare them. I want to give them more attention and love now and need to remind myself not to get caught up in other diversions.

I've often thought that the easier of the roles being played out is mine. I'm not afraid of dying. I get all sorts of love and attention. However, for those left behind there is still so much pain to get through and this saddens me greatly.

And now as I feel this way and read an earlier journal entry about "my needs not being met" I can't help but think how easy it is to be selfish.

III.

Insights Growing

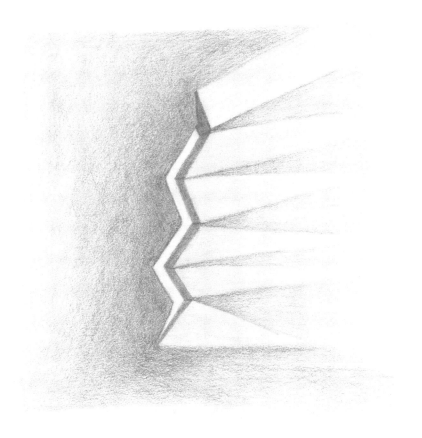

Insights Growing

Sweat in the night.
A single light shone,
Searching,
Asking,
What? Where have I gone?

Tossed in the night.
The light persisted,
Probing,
Exposing.
Who? Mind insisted.

Turned in the night.
The light was glowing,
Dreaming,
Revealing.
Why? Insights growing.

Kitchener, Ontario
February 2, 1995

Had a good visit in Sudbury. It was nice to see that Dad had improved so much in one month. Basically I rested a lot and ate a lot of Mom's great cooking.

I've had a cold (bronchitis) for the last week or so. What worries me is that I am spitting up blood. This symptom spurred me on to document the financials and got Judy and I to talk about funerals. We ended up going to see a funeral director and pre-arranged that end of things. Now we will call the priest and discuss some details with him.

On the way back from Sudbury I appreciated the beauty of the winter and wrote this little poem:

The winter sun casts
Long cool blue shadows
Of time honoured pines
On lakes blanketed
In a soft canvas
Of sparkling new snow.

Toronto, Ontario
At the airport
February 22, 1995

I visited my naturopath for an Integrated Touch session the other day. It started as normal and then she said that she was going to touch the area where I had a rash from shingles and to let her know if I was overpowered. I have no idea what she did but my body started to shake and I felt a few waves of energy flow through my body. After she stopped, it took me about five minutes to settle down. I wouldn't have believed it if it didn't happen to me.

Pat Carty came by for coffee with Judy and me. Judy commented that she is a very calm person. We had a great time chatting about different books. I showed her a number of my sculptures. She liked them, particularly the one called "Out of the Mud."

After Pat left, I meditated for a while and the whole time I felt a "presence" with me. I then turned my attention to start a visualization process and this "presence" became Jesus as my advisor. I was taken aback by this and felt intimidated.

Jesus has been coming to me in a variety of different ways over the past few weeks, i.e. the Padre Pio book from Frances Malloy, the Sermon on the Mount book by Emmett Fox. Pat gave me a book on the Aramaic teaching of Jesus, the language He used 2,000 years ago.

I was not surprised but I did feel overwhelmed at the time. Now I am getting used to the idea and starting to ask questions. One line of questioning has to do with becoming a "healer".

As I write this now I am in the airport on my way to Sudbury for a couple of days of rest and visit with my folks.

On top of a hill in Cambridge, Ontario
February 22, 1995

My Favourite Tree

Hello my old friend.
Anticipation is over.
I feel an overwhelming joy.
I said it wouldn't be so long.
Sorry.

Set against the clear blue winter sky,
I notice your fullness.
The intricate web of life.
Your simplicity.
You are beautiful.

Let me come close.
A Hug.
My arms can only - you're Huge!
You're rough.
I feel soft.

Can I sit?
Perfect fit in your roots.
Such support, trust.
We're one.
I'm gone.

I fill. With the afternoon light.
I fill. With the rustling weeds.
I fill. With the cool air up my nostrils.
I fill. With the wind's fingers on my neck.
I fill.

I rest my hands on you.
You bring me back.
I can feel your age
So many sunrises.
Sunsets.

Time to go.
I promise I'll be back.
I'll bring my friends.
One last look.
You are beautiful.

Sudbury, Ontario
February 22, 1995

As suddenly as it left, my creativity has come back. This morning I meditated at 6 a.m. and watched the sunrise. I feel a sense of peace, and yet at the same time an excitement.

In the air
February 25, 1995

French River trip #2* is meant to be. I just flew over the promised land and saw her in beautiful winter splendor. The French River's narrow run empties into the vastness of Georgian Bay through a network of webs. You can see where she joins the Pickerel and farther down the bay, the Key (where I caught a bass bigger than Mark Shea could even dream of). The French was frozen over yet I did see a couple of stretches of open water. Given everything else was frozen, one could only imagine the power running through those sections. And my eye noted paths back up the river delta for planning our trip.

This voyageur is daydreaming. Come dream with me.

* *The previous summer (1994), Dan and his "canoe buddies" had made a trip down a section of the French River and were planning another trip for the coming summer. There were times when Dan didn't believe that he'd live to see this next trip but dreaming about it gave him something to look forward to and he believed that keeping future plans alive kept him alive too. French River trip #2 was meant to be and it was on this trip that Dan discovered the sculpture of the Spiritual Warrior perched on a rock above the river. It is a photograph of this sculpture that is on the book's cover and which inspired the poem "Wanapitei Spiritual Warrior" written June 3, 1995.*

Kitchener, Ontario
March 8, 1995

The last week has been emotionally intense. Partly because I've been doing so much work on emotional and spiritual issues. I spent some time with my therapist, with Pat, and at the course on meditation trying to work some things out. The other part is due to the fact that I was told that I am to be recognized today at Manulife's Annual Employee Meeting with the John Rodger Memorial Award.* This news overwhelmed me at first, but by this morning I am now accepting the idea albeit a bit nervous about the attention and speeches. I really want to be aware and present during the presentation this afternoon.

I wrote Pat Carty a letter summarizing some of my learning over the past two or three months. Two key learnings are that meditation is about a place (a place of peace, of connectedness, of oneness that's difficult to describe in words) and that prayer is about feeling (not about repetitive words). The Lord's Prayer in Aramaic (Abwoon) has been instrumental in my learning to feel prayer through my body, through its sound and through its potentially expanded meaning.

*Each year, Manulife Financial awards one of its employees with the John Rodger Memorial Award. It is given to individuals who best exemplify, through business and community activities, the qualities of professionalism, integrity, leadership, and commitment to excellence. This award was presented to Dan, before more than 1,700 Manulife employees at the company's annual employee meeting on March 8, 1995.

Kitchener, Ontario
March 13, 1995

On Friday, Pat and I had a pretty intense session as I struggled with
this issue of becoming a "Healer". I described to her how I view myself
currently as a "builder". In the end, I accepted myself as I am and will use
my building strengths to enjoy life and further things I believe in. In
essence, I'll be more like the concept "doing by being" as described in the
book *Awakening in Time* [8] by Jacqueline Small. I will continue to grow in
healing aspects but focus it more to my own healing, and to the love and
support of those around me.

I had many insights from the book *Awakening in Time* as it laid out the
basics of the chakra system, the difference between ego and soul or the
Higher Self. The book lays out four basic steps or areas of work, namely:
meditation, inner or spiritual work, study and outer work or service. Last
week I had much clarity on the first two.

Going forward, I will increase my level of study and while I will
continue to keep the influence as broad as possible, I sense that my study
should focus on Jesus. In terms of outer work or service, I will use my
strengths as I have done in the Canadian Cancer Society business campaign
as I lay a foundation for future campaigns, influence the direction of
marketing at Manulife in order to be customer-focused, continue my
artwork as a form of expression and as a joy of working with my hands...
I think I'll also brainstorm building in other ways like building awareness
of cancer patients' needs.

Forks of the Credit
March 28, 1995

I sit by the Forks of the Credit River listening to the sound of water and feeling the sun on my face. I dropped in on Judy's uncle, Jim Lyons, at the farm for lunch and a beer. Great to see Jim; he is so supportive.

Had a good time up at Collingwood and I really needed to get away with Judy and the kids. I was wound up pretty tight, I think because I've been running myself too hard. I get grumpy and edgy when I'm tired.

Mike Burke was down Friday night for the film Waterwalker[9] and spent until Saturday at 4:30 before he headed home. We had a good time.

By The Credit

The water passes by
Just like time.
I close my eyes
And hear the water in its fullness.
I know I can't stop the water,
Nor can I stop time.

As I Am

I am not worthy.
I am not unworthy.
I am.

Jesus love me.

Jesus love me.
I'll love others as best as I can.

God love me.

God love me,
And I'll love others as I am.

Kitchener, Ontario
April 18, 1995

Things have been going well. Actually a bit tough on the physical side as I have had a lot of coughing over the past week. Things are going well with Judy and I as we seem to both be coping well and have patience for each other. Mom, Dad and Marilyn were down for Easter and that was a good weekend overall. But I was tired by the end of it.

I am doing a 12-week course in a book called *The Artist's Way* [10] which has me journaling three pages a day plus doing certain exercises. I'm enjoying it. Judy started today.

Got a whole new insight into goal setting. Rather than my old way with three, six, twelve month plus lifetime goals I am working on daily practises in goal areas.

Goal Areas/Values	**Daily Practises**
Spiritual Growth	Prayer - the Light Invocation Meditation Contemplation Study
Healing Self	Rest Exercise, Walk Eat Well Emotional Release Creativity (art) *The Artist's Way* which includes journaling and artist date
Relationships	Spend Time Awareness, Courage and Gentleness Balance between letting go and holding on
Service to Others	Volunteering with Canadian Cancer Society and HopeSpring Contribute at work Raise awareness Support other cancer friends

Kitchener, Ontario
April 23, 1995

Just Do It

Man, 45, watches another TV ad. A young man running in bright white sneakers. And the slogan brags, "Just do it."

Young man, 20, in a war. Another one of the guys. Not really so bad. Complains, "But there are women and children." Order, "Just do it."

Years earlier, young boy on the farm. Another long day. Friends far away. He's sad. Says, "Dad, can I stop now and go play?" Father yells, "Just do it."

Men, many men, throughout life when there may be a choice to be had, may want to stop, think, talk, feel. But the inner critic shouts, "Just do it."

Kitchener, Ontario
May 29, 1995

Obsessed

Attention, affection, intimacy,
I am obsessed with these
And can't let them go.
All I have to do is ask,
But I don't ask.
I am wanting to be free,
But unwilling to be free.
Such a paradox
To be obsessed.

Wanapitei Spiritual Warrior

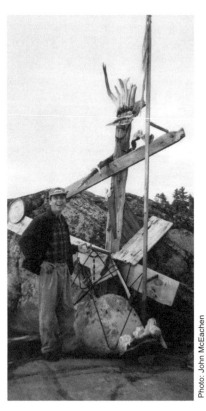

Photo: John McEachen

Dan, standing beside the "sculpture"
that he and his canoe buddies
discovered on their June '95 trip along
the French River.

What a find!
You are so wonderful, fun, fantastic.
I am like a child around you,
gazing in wonder and delight.
Boards, rocks, axes, springs,
saws, driftwood, chains, rocks
and a fishing pole -
talk about a multimedia sculpture.

And you are so appropriately titled
Spiritual Warrior.

Spirituality is built the same way you are.
In bits and pieces.
Old wounds and scars, discarded,
used and sometimes abused pasts.
Pieces carved out of time
like the driftwood that is your crown.
The rocks, your foundation,
have just always been there.
Yet someone did take the time
to painstakingly put you together.
Not only with bolts and nails,
but with enthusiasm and care
to make you sturdy.

Spirituality is a lonely quest.
Alone on this barren rock.
Standing tall
through the fiercest storms.
Braving guard
in the darkest night.
But look at you now.
Basking in this glorious sunset.
Look at your view now.
The angels of yellow and purple dance
on the clouds for you.
Enjoy, oh spiritual warrior.

Thank you for the joy
you have given to me.

Kitchener, Ontario
June 12, 1995

Learning

As I pass through
A thought will enter,
"And what did you learn?"

The rustling leaves
Flutter to the ground
Providing a warm blanket for new growth.

The majestic tree
Lays down peacefully
So a seedling can burst forth in new life.

Truest intentions
Resonate through space
To spawn the new light for loving action.

Kitchener, Ontario
June 23, 1995

In The Moment

Look around you.
This is all there is.
This too is everything.
For in the sparkling water,
In the bird's song,
Lives the spirit.

Kitchener, Ontario
June 24, 1995

Quite a day yesterday. Pat Carty and I went to Schneider's farm for a walk. I brought along one of the Essene books* and we read a poem called "The most ancient revelation" as we started out.

I speak to you.
Be Still
Know
I Am
God

This is an excellent mantra for a walking meditation because as you say it, it reminds you to stop. Then you see, hear, smell the wonders. We walked to the top of a hill and did a reading from Book One on the Angel of Air, Water and Sun.[11] It was a simply wonderful experience standing on the hill with a slight breeze and sun shining brightly.

I see Pat as my teacher, my spiritual teacher. She complimented me by saying she learns from me and called me her spiritual friend. It really is nice to have a spiritual friend, someone to talk to openly about my doubts, confusion, learning and to share insights that I get from reading different books.

* *The Essenes lived in spiritual communities that existed in the deserts of the Middle East well over 2,000 years ago. They were dedicated to preserving the ancient teachings. Discovery of the Dead Sea Scrolls in 1947 brought to new light the wisdom-teachings of the Essene communities. They lived in simple harmony with all of nature which is what appealed to Dan.*

Hilltop Memory

Standing upon a hilltop,
In the sunlight,
Complete in prayer from the soul.

Driven not by coincidence,
By an instinct,
By a memory of the soul.

Hearts expanded to heaven,
And did create
A new memory in my soul.

In the afternoon I went for a massage. My massage therapist is a wonderful and compassionate person. I find that I open up to her quickly and she is very wise. I left there feeling extremely relaxed and at peace.

Judy and I went to see the movie "Bridges of Madison County"[12] in the evening. It is a very moving and passionate love story. It rekindled in me many of the passions I have in me that I have also buried more than once. I could empathize with Francesca in her desire/dream for an all-out passionate love. I have felt that in the past, but during the last two-and-a-half years since my illness I have had to deal with letting go. During April and May I journaled about a lot of my feelings around these issues and then after the canoe trip I burned these journals in a ritual of letting them go. I have been at peace with this since, but the movie certainly touched these wounds.

I have always been a passionate man. I loved food, wine, work, play, love, sex, and touch all with great enthusiasm. I still carry this passion in me but because of diet, sex and energy restraints I have learned to live with them differently. Also I've made a spiritual change, have grown tremendously in my understanding of God, nature, self, mind and spirit (especially in the last six months, coached by Pat). As a result, the passion is changing more to compassion. In other words, less on my own needs, especially physical passions, and more on the emotional and spiritual needs of both myself and others.

My basic enthusiasm for life is still there, and actually very strong, just directed differently. It is different and I think more fulfilling as I feel the connectedness with others now, as well as a sort of timelessness with "others". I also feel a deeper level of love, a great ocean of it, from many sources.

So in one day I cycle through spirit, body, passion, and this morning brings another day of exploring, surprises, changes, experience and love.

IV.

Dying

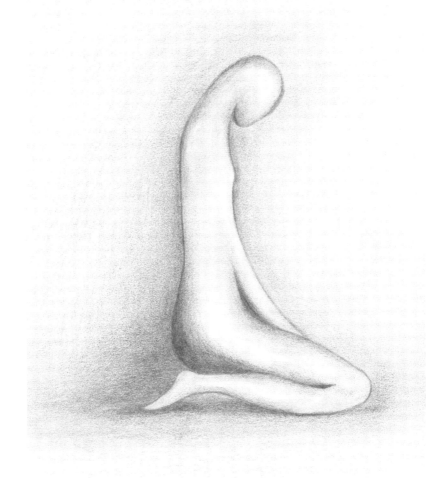

Kitchener, Ontario
June 25, 1995

Home

I grieve
The loss of this body.

I mourn
The death of this tree.

Both were home to me.

Hands
(To my Dad)

Me
I feel
The hard edges of stone,
Slippery wetness of fish,
Delicate lightness of feather,
Rough scales of this tree.

You.
Remember
Your strength holding me up,
Expressive gestures fluently speaking,
Gentleness with seed to earth,
Stern delivery of a needed message.

Hands
Watch them.
Poised to sign in war and peace,
Quickly moving in games of life,
Dancing high in full moon's light,
Folded in prayer of mourning.

God
Creator's hand.
Giver of robust and abundant beauty,
Nurturer of the spirit of freedom,
Comforter of the aching lonely soul,
Always.

Sculpted in the tree.

Kitchener, Ontario
June 26, 1995

Rhythm

I feel life
Surging
Through me.
Rhythm.
Baby suckling.
Lovers pulsating.
Monks chanting.

Kitchener, Ontario
June 27, 1995

Alive

I am going to grieve
While I live,
So I can be alive
When I die.

Kitchener, Ontario
June 29, 1995

Pour My Ashes On The River

Pour my ashes on the river,
Let me run free and wild.
Someday I'll come thundering down,
Taming Africa's roaring wild.
Some night, flushing down,
Swirling, jazz, rhythm of the soul.
Pour my ashes on the river
Freedom for all, for soul.

No Anger Here

There'll be no anger in this house,
Not male anger in any case.
Or anything that even looks
Smells, feels, sounds like it.
None.

It finds its way out though,
When least expected.
Other emotions get manipulated
Squashed, distorted, exaggerated by it.
Ooo-aahh.

Its confusion then rebounds through
the house for days on end.
Everything keeps getting bounced,
Banged, bumped, busted by it.
Boom.

When all seems well, settled,
There waits the hidden coal,
All too ready to spark
Flame, crackle, ROAR for it.
ANGER.

My Spirituality

Reading about spiritual leaders,
Gurus, lamas, priests and such,
At times, awed and inspired
And then, puzzled and discouraged,
Not sure I want that life much.

Amazed by their rigorous discipline,
Continuous devotion,
Days on end in their pose.
I have trouble sitting still
For a brief meditation.

From time to time there comes big news
A vision, a signal, God
The word spreads like wildfire
And devotees flock together
Longing for a prayed-for nod.
My spirituality is here, now,
In body, mind, soul, in one,
Trust it for eternity.

Port Elgin, Ontario
At Mike Burke's cottage
July 10, 1995

Blue

Deep blue water
Where it meets the horizon
moody blue above
thoughts of you
My head falls back
into the chaise chair
witnessing the oppressive gray
clouds hanging low
A gray gull wanders
never seen one so confused
searching left, right, up, down
ah, it's found a direction
I lose it in the gray
Pick up the treeline
shoreline
waveline
momentarily lost
soothing motion
soft brown sand
footprints
thoughts of you.

Simple Pleasures

Boy and grandpa
laughing by the stream.
"Born and raised in Alberta
Ya know
wasn't much to do.
So we caught
frogs and things."

Swish with net,
frog panics about.
"A real wopper.
Like to take the boys
out like this,
learn something
a real experience,
ya know."

Boy watching, touching
the wopper in the
bottom of a green pond.
Whispers Grandpa
"Couldn't make 'em
happier with a
million dollars.
Ya know."

Smile.
Smile.
Wide-mouthed smile.

Port Elgin, Ontario
July 12, 1995

I read a poem called "In the Beginning was the Word" from *The Collected Poems of Al Purdy*. [13] I was sitting on a rock jutting out from the shore at Mike Burke's cottage today. The poem motivated me to really listen to all the sounds around me and to imitate them as early man did in the development of speech. I had one of those "ah-ha" experiences while imitating the sound of the wind blowing face on. Sounded like "oooo" in "abwoon" and so I came to understand the reading on "abwoon" in the book *Prayers of the Cosmos* [14] by Neil Douglas-Klotz and to understand the ancients in the Aum or Ohm chants. I felt a connectedness through time. As the poem ends, "And the children remembered."

Port Elgin, Ontario
July 12, 1995

Common Beings

Four common terns
turn in unison
around the rocky shore
then break formation
as each homes
in on a landing
at water's edge
they sit I watch
I watch they sit
they watch I sit
common beings
being.

Flame Eternal

My torch burns for you.
Flame eternal.

No storm, wild stuff.
No wave, large enough.
Fiercely held so high.
Universal.

All paths, farthest away,
All night, all day.

My torch burns for you.

Sacred Love

You know I'll be back,
Some time, some place,
I'll know you, you me,
Both blessed with grace.
Twinkle in your eye,
Wonder in your face,
A moment will hang in the air,
Breathe into that, that space,
Knowing it is our love,
Vibrating in a sacred place.

Kitchener, Ontario
July 25, 1995

To write poetry,
You really have to be alone.
To be alone,
You really had to have been with somebody.

Kitchener, Ontario
July 26, 1995

Hunched Over

Sunlight casts ever-changing shadows through the trees
as I hunched over, eyes open wide
letting out a series of very low staccato grunts
so keen so tuned so sensing this animal
no wonder the ingenious predator developed.
Weapon in hand fondling then zeroing in on a ripple
peak tension buzzing alertness forceful ripping grip
quietly sneaking plotting a path of death
moistening in anticipation a special nighttime reward
a shape not a tree or stump a prey locked in fear
no fear here a hunger for survival a kill
a strong pulsing beat inside so loud the kill.
All is quiet breath light wisps mixed with wind
a smile joins a different drum that now beats inside
bumbumbum Boom Boom - bumbumbum Boom Boom
a dance will erupt tonight in thanks
bumbumbum Boom Boom - bumbumbum Boom Boom.

Miracles

I looked in the phone book under miracles,
Miracle Food Mart, Miracle Pools, Miracle Water.
I dialed 1-800-MIRACLE (647-2253).
Electric Ma Bell "This number is not in service".
And then a voice popped into my head,
An old Jewish male, don't ask me why.
"What, you're looking for a miracle.
I'll tell you what. Open your eyes.
There are miracles all around you."
Oh yeah, I've been down that road before,
The flowering trees, the singing birds
The birthing baby, the rising sun,
But this ain't what I need. I need
A real, outright, amazing, cure-type miracle.
"You, who are so lucky to have been born,
Let me tell you, it's a miracle that you'll die.
What do you think would happen
If we all lived on this earth forever?"
Um, a tough question, but an exception
now and again, would it be so bad?
"Well, now you're talking about the law.
Beg and grovel all you want for a miracle,
It won't happen, it just won't happen.
But then sometimes, there comes a miracle
And then you'll say to yourself 'This really is a miracle'
So don't worry, don't look, don't wait, listen to me
Listen to me. You are a miracle. That's all I have to say.
Good-bye." The old Jew is gone, I close up the phone book,
Pick up my coffee cup, Ummm. Thank God for small miracles.

The Spirit Of My Dove

I am sculpture.
I am the sculptor,
I create form in space.

I am a dance.
I am the dancer,
I float, body and face.

I am a song.
I am a singer,
I celebrate with love.

I am created.
I am creator,
The spirit of my dove.

Kitchener, Ontario
August 11, 1995

My ultimate goal, my released dove, is to die in peace. I think this means continuing my spiritual practices and growth. I have been sloppy lately with the consistency of my practices. I feel Judy and I are on the right path. I need to spend a bit more quality time with the boys.

HopeSpring is important to me and for me in terms of my growth, keeping active and fulfilling my current purpose of building awareness.

Is the outcome of my human body my soul's choice? I have heard this. OK, I suppose it is. But how much influence do I have over my soul and this decision? I've been fighting hard and stretching time and quality but I could do more I'm sure. Or can I accept my death, which I have, and continue to share my creativity, emotions as Bernie Siegal says, "play the important role of the wounded soldier." I feel a oneness that I've never felt before. Even my poem, "The Spirit of My Dove" shows this continuum from the manifested body to the spirit that I believe in and feel. So I should listen to the body for clues and I should listen to all parts in between.

Kitchener, Ontario
August 20, 1995

Had a good visit to Sudbury. Just long enough to connect but I was exhausted yesterday and am tired out today. Had a good visit with my mother. We went for a walk up at Mario and Mary's cottage for an hour and she opened up a bit. The next day we talked some more. It's very hard for them to accept this situation. I feel good that I was open and supportive.

Kitchener, Ontario
August 21, 1995

I had a really bad day yesterday. Frustrated with my physical limitations. Angry and sad about the current situation. I think I was emotionally drained, still tired and then blew up at Michael. Feel a bit better today but must pace myself. Start 714X (an experimental cancer treatment) today — that's positive and I intend to make the most of it.

Kitchener, Ontario
August 21, 1995

Rage

You know you're ready to write
when you desperately grab pen and paper
and hurl all over it.
The shit just pours out,
anger reddens, ink pain oozes out.
Then piece it back together slowly,
word by word put it back together.
Thought by thought words laboured with will,
until you feel the release, a sigh,
as the pen silently lifts off the paper
with the last word.

Kitchener, Ontario
September 2, 1995

My cousin Giulianna's husband, Omero, died in a car accident a week ago today. He was found the next day dead in a ditch. What a tragedy. Poor Giulianna, Marina and Eva. Poor Zio Dino and Zia Nida. They've not yet recovered from Sandro's death last year.* They must be in great pain. God help them.

It's been two weeks now that I have been emotionally burned out. And physically, with my shortness of breath, I am able to do less and less and this tends to frustrate me.

I'm slowly rebuilding again though. The videos by Father Bede Griffith[15] were insightful — God as eternity, the unlimited, the unknowing, the mystery manifested through the word, man, Jesus and willed by love, goodness through the spirit. He does this summary in a way that pulls all the great religions together.

I watched a video about Gabrielle Roth called "I Dance the Body Electric"[16] and liked the part when she says, "... and then you realize that there is no perfect answer, no one way, no dogma to cover your ass . . . you are at the edge, let everything go, move into the emptiness and shift from the ego to the soul." She says the three "I's" of the soul are Intuition, Imagination, and Inspiration. Inspiration is the food of the soul. The ego desires food from the culture, i.e., sex, cars, popcorn. The soul hungers for a different thing. It hungers for inspiration.

Man, do I want to get to my tree soon.**

---

* *Dan and I had been in Italy during the summer of 1992 with our sons Dennis and Michael and Dan's sister Marilyn. We stayed with relatives in a small village in the north of Italy where Dan's parents come from. Zio Dino, Dan's uncle, is the only sibling of Dan's mother. He had two children, Dan's first cousins. Guilianna, the oldest, born a year after Dan, was married to Omero. Sandro was in his early thirties and when we were in Italy was planning his wedding to Elena. Shortly after we came home, after a fabulous trip spent with wonderful people, Dan was diagnosed with cancer; a year later Sandro was killed in a car accident and a month before Dan died, Giulianna's husband, Omero, was also killed in a car accident. Marina and Eva are the children of Giulianna and Omero.*

** *See Dan's poem, "My Favourite Tree" (February 22, 1995)*

Kitchener, Ontario
September 10, 1995

Energy and breathing have been very poor over the last two days. Emotionally I am very vulnerable and crying a lot. I am having trouble letting go.

Kitchener, Ontario
September 11, 1995

Last night was just an emotional disaster for me. I couldn't stop crying, feeling so depressed and unable to let it go.

Kitchener, Ontario
September 21, 1995

Grateful for the support and friendship that Pat gave me the other day. She really has a way of helping me discover the real questions and strive for the greater truths. I couldn't believe how much better I felt physically after our discussion. I have turned the corner emotionally although letting go is easier said than done.

Kitchener, Ontario
September 22, 1995

The Sudbury trip went well for me and my parents. I broke the pattern I was into and I felt much more even-keeled the last couple of days. Pat's talk before I went north helped a lot. My breathing is very poor and I think I've had enough of the morphine. Oh well.

Kitchener, Ontario
September 26, 1995

Felt really poorly so I called Aerocare *(a company that provides home oxygen and equipment)*. The oxygen flow had to be increased considerably which meant new equipment. This has made a real difference.

I also called my palliative care physician who came by and decided we needed to get ahead of the pain. She ordered a pain pump, changed some meds, ordered an electric bed and I'm feeling a whole lot better.

Swept Up High

Swept up high in the grass
Floating like two spirit forms,
A dance
So free and graceful,
That tears could not be held back.

Each sparkling tear drop
Flung with rhythmic pleasure,
Chose a perfect note
So clear and wonderful,
That song erupted in ecstasy.

The song spiraled out
Weaving a mystical love
Inspired the dancers and tears
To give all their heart,
Free and timeless as cosmic art.

Kitchener, Ontario
September 27, 1995

The pain pump and electric bed certainly have made a difference. I had a decent sleep last night. Now to pace myself. Foot swelling has been bad and breathing showing very little improvement.

Kitchener, Ontario
September 28, 1995

Worked like a dog today, mostly on HopeSpring stuff. Had a lot of work but definitely burned myself out. Going to bed has been a DRUG WAR.

Kitchener, Ontario
September 29, 1995

Quite another action-packed day today with VON *(Victorian Order of Nurses who provide home nursing care)*, Aerocare, and lots of visitors. It's 5:30 and other than a little pain in my leg, I'm hanging in. Judy is needing peace and quiet for sure. I'll bring this up tonight or tomorrow and see what we can figure out in terms of controlled vs. non-controlled visits.

Kitchener, Ontario
October 4, 1995

About The Unresolved

This fall the black cherry tree will change
its colour for the last time.
As the season comes to a close its bright
offerings will both be danced and gently
added to the mosaic floor or
blown ragingly in a fierce battle that
will chill you to the bone.
And you see there before you
those last yellow and brown leaves
that will stay and hug night after night.
Some are issues
not resolved.
Some are forgivenesses
not given.
Some are regrets
stubbornly retained,
Mostly human
not to be perfected.

In time. . . .
The odd issue not resolved
mostly didn't matter anyway.
Those forgivenesses not given
were not really meant to be forgiven
from within,
But it was understood
that they were to be forgiven
from without.
The regrets, so stubborn over time,
look completely different when
reframed from the other side.
Some humans, not perfect,
will stand back to take time
in the wonder and beauty of it all.

*This final poem was finished on Wednesday evening, October 4. Dan Blasutti died at
6:30 a.m. on Thursday, October 5, 1995 at home. He died fully conscious and in peace as
he wished.*

99

AFTERWORD

Very soon after I met Dan Blasutti, he asked me to help him die. At a very soul level I knew I was being offered a precious gift and was touched by his request. I was also afraid. Although I had studied and practiced yoga, meditation and visualization for years and had taught and worked with many people with cancer, I had never been with anyone as they died. My main spiritual practice is the Divine Light Invocation but I had never yet guided anyone into Light not to return. Yet I had faith that God never asks us to do something we are not ready to do.

Dan said he wanted to die with spiritual awareness and was worried that he would not be able to keep focused on the spiritual practices that he and I had been working on together. He accepted that he would not escape his physical death but wanted to be fully present to all of life's moments as they came. The student/teacher relationship that developed between us began after I agreed to help Dan recover his meditative practice, something he lost because of an increased need for morphine as his cancer progressed.

After I agreed to help him, the relationship moved into much deeper territory. Masks were quickly stripped away and a sacred bond developed between us. Dying is a very intimate time, emotions are raw, exposed. The year I spent with Dan as his teacher and his friend was intense, challenging and rewarding.

My role was not really to "teach" Dan anything but to guide him to uncover his own inner wisdom and clarify his own beliefs. One of the main precepts of the yogic tradition is that the teacher not take the joy of self-discovery from a student. It was in this way that I worked with Dan and because of his insatiable curiosity it was a joy to watch.

He eagerly read and studied everything I suggested, wrote papers and letters, continually defining and expanding his understanding. We worked with prayer, symbolism, ritual. In the process of living his dying and in his ever-deepening search for purpose and meaning, Dan challenged me to bring forth all my training.

At one point he was struggling with the Lord's Prayer, finding he could not focus on the words. I suggested studying it in its original language, Aramaic, from a book called *Prayers of the Cosmos* by Neil Douglas-Klotz. Dan not only studied it but memorized it completely. Reciting it in this new way allowed him to experience its deeper meaning. We walked, talked, laughed, cried. It was a co-mingling of souls, a holy offering, a sacred loving communion. The night before Dan died, I felt blessed to be with him. All who were there agree we witnessed something truly magical. The spiritual practices Dan had integrated over the past year came easily and naturally to him that night. It was a time of pure awareness, breath by breath, moment by moment.

When Dan died, some part of me died too. But also what died was my fear of dying. Underlying his pain and my sense of loss was an awakening of a vibrant appreciation that dying can bring forth something mystical and that each moment of life is precious and not to be wasted.

After they had taken Dan's body away, I placed a long-stemmed red rose on his bed. This was for me a final gesture of love, admiration and respect for this special being. The rose symbolized his journey of life and death — the stem being the path, the thorns the sharpness and pain, the exquisite flower, the pearl of great price. Hari Om.

Pat Carty

Notes

1. Cohen, Leonard. Excerpt from the poem "Anthem," in Stranger Music, Selected Poems and Songs (Toronto: McClelland & Stewart, Inc., 1993), p. 373.

2. Frankl, Viktor Emil. Man's Search for Meaning: an introduction to Logotherapy (Boston: Beacon Press)

3. Siegel, Bernie S. Peace, Love & Healing (New York: Harper & Row, Publishers, Inc., 1989)

4. Chopra, Deepak. Quantum Healing, Exploring the Frontiers of Mind/BodyMedicine (New York: Bantam Books, 1989)

5. Ramljak, Suzanne. "Interview with Donald Saff," in Sculpture, November/December 1994 (Washington, D.C.: International Sculpture Centre), pp 10-12.

6. Harper, Tom. "The Creative Spirit," in God Help Us (Toronto: McClelland & Stewart, Inc., 1992), pp 88-90.

7. Radha, Swami Sivananda. The Divine Light Invocation (Spokane, Washington: Timeless Books, 1990)

8. Small, Jacqueline. Awakening in Time: the journey from co-dependence to co-creation (New York, Toronto: Bantam Books, 1991)

9. Waterwalker, produced by Bill Mason, National Film Board of Canada, 1985.

10. Cameron, Julia. The Artist's Way, A Spiritual Path to Higher Creativity (New York: G.P. Putnam's Sons, 1992)

11. Szekely, Edmond Bordeaux, ed. and translator. The Essene Gospel of Peace, Book One and Book Two. (Matsqui, British Columbia, Canada: The International Biogenic Society)

12. Bridges of Madison County, with Clint Eastwood and Meryl Streep, Warner Brothers, 1995

13. Brown, Russell, ed. "In the Beginning was the Word," in The Collected Poems of Al Purdy (Toronto: McClelland & Stewart, Inc., 1989 edition), p. 299.

14. Douglas-Klotz, Neil. Prayers of the Cosmos (New York: Harper & Row Publishers, 1990)

15. Griffith, Father Bede. Books, tapes and other work by Father Bede Griffith are available from Incarnation Monastery, c/o Br. Cassian Hardie, OSB Cam., 1369 La Loma Ave., Berkeley, CA 94708.

16. I Dance the Body Electric. Video of an interview with Gabrielle Roth available from The Moving Centre, P.O. Box 070, Redbank, New Jersey.

Index of Poetry

PERMISSIONS